Apple Cider Vinegar
CLEANSE

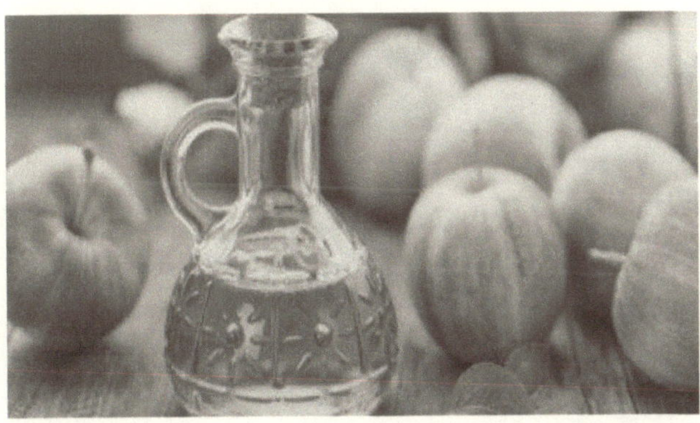

"Jump Start Your Metabolism, Enjoy Natural Weight Loss and Enhance Whole Body Health with This Ancient Miracle Supplement"

Dana Lee

Apple Cider Vinegar Cleanse

Published by:

Dana Publishing
P.O. Box 1801
Mentor, OH 44060

Legal & Disclaimer

The information contained in this book and its contents is not designed to replace or take the place of any form of medical or professional advice; and is not meant to replace the need for independent medical, financial, legal or other professional advice or services, as may be required. The content and information in this book has been provided for educational and entertainment purposes only.

The content and information contained in this book has been compiled from sources deemed reliable, and it is accurate to the best of the Author's knowledge, information and belief. However, the Author cannot guarantee its accuracy and validity and cannot be held liable for any errors and/or omissions. Further, changes are periodically made to this book as and when needed. Where appropriate and/or necessary, you must consult a professional (including but not limited to your doctor, attorney, financial advisor or such other professional advisor) before using any of the suggested remedies, techniques, or information in this book.

Upon using the contents and information contained in this book, you agree to hold harmless the Author from and against any damages, costs, and expenses, including any legal fees potentially resulting from the application of any of the information provided by this book. This disclaimer applies to any loss, damages or injury caused by the use and application, whether directly or indirectly, of any advice or information presented, whether for breach of contract, tort, negligence, personal injury, criminal intent, or under any other cause of action.

You agree to accept all risks of using the information presented inside this book.

You agree that by continuing to read this book, where appropriate and/or necessary, you shall consult a professional (including but not limited to your doctor, attorney, or financial advisor or such other advisor as needed) before using any of the suggested remedies, techniques, or information in this book.

Table of Contents

Introduction

There is a favorite dressing ingredient used for salad: that ingredient is Apple Cider Vinegar. However, it is also marketed as a natural remedy. It is believed to help to reduce weight, dandruff, constipation, and treat conditions like diabetes and cancer. But do these health claims have scientific evidence, and is apple cider vinegar safe?

Apple cider vinegar is usually apple juice, but adding yeast will turn the sugar in the liquid into alcohol. This is called the fermentation process. Bacteria convert alcohol into acetic acid. That is what makes the taste of vinegar sour and strong.

Apple vinegar has been treating conditions such as sore neck and varicose veins for many years. The claims are not supported by much science. In recent years, however, some researchers have looked closer to the potential benefits of apple cider vinegar.

Many claim that the "mother" -the cloud of yeast and bacteria that can be contained in an apple cider vinegar bottle- is what makes it safe. Such products contain probiotics, which means that they can improve the digestive system, but there is not enough evidence to support these claims.

You may have a friend who wants to take fat burning shots of apple cider vinegar at night. Or, in the refrigerated food shop, you may have seen apple cider vinegar beverages. With this seemingly essential liquid's explosive success, you probably wonder what the benefits and uses are.

Let's first explore what Apple Cider Vinegar, or ACV, is precisely. ACV consists of fermented apples and water. As with other kinds of vinegar, ACV has 5% acidity.

You can note that stores carry different types of ACVs. For example, distilled ACV looks bright in the bottle, and it may be the one you know best. Nevertheless, untreated, unfiltered, and unpasteurized ACV contains a dark material floating in the mixture. This is called "mother," and is formed during fermentation by natural enzymes. No need to be careful about it: this fibrous material usually sinks to the bottom of the bottle, is consumable and absolutely safe.

Whatever the type, you don't have to refrigerate ACV, and it will last a very long time. According to The Vinegar Institute, a **global trade association for vinegar manufacturers**, *Vinegar generally has an almost indefinite shelf life*. Even if your vinegar changes appearance (for example, it may look more cloudy), it's still all right to be used. Apple cider vinegar has been a staple in the kitchen for decades, but few have known its active uses over and above splashing on a salad or a dash in a dish. The raw, unfiltered form of ACV is very different from the regular apple cider vinegar on almost every food store shelf. How vinegar is produced is the difference between the organic and unfiltered variants and the highly processed version. Organically, apple vinegar is more nutritious and has more significant health benefits. When looking at them, the distinction between organic and non-organic cider vinegar can be seen physically. Organic ACV appears to be somewhat dark, with bottled water at the bottom. Any visible, non-organic ACV particles are bright. This is because the non-organic material is pasteurized— a method in which a product is heated and distilled. The pasteurization process removes many of the bacteria, nutrients, and enzymes that occur naturally in apple cider vinegar – commonly known as the 'mom.'

As far as health facts are concerned, you should rest assured that ACV does have any per se. Diluted apple cider vinegar does not contain any calories per tablespoon, nor fat, carbohydrates, protein, or sugar. You can see that as an excellent way to add an explosion of flavor to your food without adding calories or extra salt.

Apple cider vinegar (ACV) has actually been utilized for thousands of years. From the ancient Babylonians to the Romans, everyone used this as a cure for all sorts of health problems.

Like coconut oil and grass-fed butter, ACV comes back to healthy individuals.

Regardless of where you look, you will find someone who makes wild claims on what ACV can do for their health, appearance, and home. Many arguments are historical, and scientific research has not confirmed them...yet. But many other cases have been tested and proven scientifically.

Keep reading if you want to learn how ACV can help you.

Chapter 1:
What is Apple Cider Vinegar?

Apple vinegar is made from fermented apple juice converted by specific bacteria into vinegar. Apple cider vinegar has a mild and crisp flavor with the compounds in apples. Other foods can be made into vinegar, such as grapes, oranges, bananas, maple syrup, grains, and even beer. They all have their own unique flavors.

ACV is a salty, acidic (you guessed it) apple water!

It is a two-stage process: manufacturers first expose broken apples to yeast. In a process called fermentation, the sugar is absorbed by the yeast and converted into alcohol.

The producers also add acid-forming bacteria (i.e., acetobacter) to further alcohol fermentation. It then transforms into a liquid called "acetic acid," the major component of ACV. This bacterium converts the ethanol into vinegar. Acetic acid and malic acid give vinegar's acid flavor to apple cider.

Apple Cider Vinegar (ACV) is a yeast-fermented apple cider.

It's vinegar. Although it is possible to produce vinegar with a wide variety of carbohydrates, apples are the only source of the unique health benefits and taste of this vinegar.

Some ingredients for apple cider were just as hyped as vinegar.

Scarlett Johansson says that washing her face with distilled apple cider vinegar keeps her skin clear. Explorer Sir Ranulph Fiennes swears by this, saying that he was battling arthritis with a daily snack drink.

Apple Cider Vinegar Nutrition Facts

Cider vinegar (ACV) contains only a few calories but packs an enormous nutritional punch. While ACV does contain traces of iron and potassium, it does not contain many vitamins or minerals.

Vinegar (organic, or non-pasteurized) also includes protein strings, enzymes, and beneficial bacteria (i.e., probiotics). The ingredients are contained in a cobweb-like substance known as "mommy." The mother is 100 percent edible, typically floating at the bottom of ACV containers.

Acetic acid itself, as well as unpasteurized ACV enzymes and other minerals, provide the most nutritional benefits.

Apple cider vinegar (ACV) is a popular condiment and health food. It is made from apples by fermenting it with live plants, minerals, and acids.

As a home remedy, ACV has many uses. One of these is as a hair wash to improve the health of your scalp, strengthen your skin, and improve its shine.

Although it is praised as a "panacea" or "cure-all" for health problems, the advantages, and the science behind ACV can aid in hair care in particular.

Apple cider vinegar can be an excellent natural remedy to try for those with hair problems, such as itchy scalp and hair breakage.

Wouldn't it just be incredible to have a secret potion to perfect it all? For years I have thought of a beautiful product or food that can be multifunctional. Everything that can treat my hair and skin correctly can keep me healthy and fit to help out my mother with some of the necessary household tasks. Vinegar is something that can be used very well. Sadly, we are not big vinegar fans in India. As compared to Western food fans, we generally use less vinegar in our everyday cooking. We are less familiar with the fantastic, magical properties and the value of vinegar as a daily salad dressing hit than those used to many European, Asian, and Western cuisines.

The most common vinegar in the natural health community is Apple Cider Vinegar. The use in the West has undergone a growing trend, while in India, it remains relatively less used. Apple cider vinegar is extracted after extensive processing and fermentation of apple pulp. This elixir has many advantages: from promising lustrous hair and flawless skin to avoiding health risks, and the ultimate help in solving some of your toughest household chores. Look at what makes this cocktail so amazing.

Chapter 2:
The History of Apple Cider Vinegar

Vinegar was likely a happy accident, created separately in different parts of the world; a bottle of wine or beer was too long uncovered, and a culinary legend was born. The legacy of vinegar dates back at least 8000 years; vessels with vinegar traces dating from 6000 B.C.E were found in Egypt and China.

It is reported that around 5,000 B.C.E. that the Babylonians used vinegar made with dates as a preservative and a condiment, and they started experimenting with aromatic kinds of vinegar using herbs and spices. While the usefulness of vinegar in the kitchen has been known for thousands of years, the first to prescribe vinegar for a range of diseases and preventive needs was Hippocrates (around 400 B.C.E.).

Hippocrates had long been known to use apple cider vinegar as a tonic for health. Since then, home remedy books and old maid's tales have all prescribed the treatment of this vinegar. Dr. Jarvis wrote a book in 1958 on the health benefits of apple cider. According to his instructions, cider vinegar should be mixed with sweet honey, and a teaspoon should be taken every day. By the 1970s, the popularity of apple cider vinegar had increased again. After reading his book, the proponents were used to create an apple cider vinegar weight loss plan.

Some remnants of apple cider vinegar found in a vase dating back to pre-Pharaonic times were found in Egypt, indicating that Egyptians were aware of it and used it to preserve food, just as the people of Babylon and Persia did. Vinegar can be used to carry food on long journeys. Mixed with water, farmers and travelers used it in ancient times to quench thirst.

Vinegar for disease and other health conditions has been used since the time of Hippocrates (roughly 460–377 B.C.). A Greek medical practitioner, known as the "father of medicine," used vinegar to purify injuries and to treat open and infected lacerations, and also prescribed a vinegar and honey combination for chronic respiratory conditions.

The "Mother" in Apple Cider Vinegar

Apple cider vinegar includes an all-powerful "mother," the sediment-like and cobweb-like material which can be seen in unfiltered ACV products. The mother contains concentrated bacteria and enzymes that make ACV so well known for its antifungal, antiviral, and anti-bacterial healing properties. Although some people can be put off ACV bottles by the water, this component is the product of special processing that preserves apple nutrients and enzymes during the fermentation process and thus offers specific curative powers for the ACV.

From Babylonians to Samurai Warriors

Vinegar is one of the oldest fermentation methods known to man, from Ancient Babylonians to samurai warriors. The earliest process of fermentation is wine from which the first vinegar had been made. The Babylonians, dated back to 5000 BC, made date palm wine, while the Egyptians made barley wine. Around 2500 BC, an ancient nomadic tribe called the Aryans made a sour wine from apples and this is considered to be a precursor for the cider. The word 'cider' is derived from the Phoenician 'Shekar,' which means wine or strong drink. So from the Babylonians, the Aryans, the Phoenicians, the Greeks, and the Romans got the soiled apple wine recipe, and people began to develop Apple cider vinegar as a byproduct of their soiled apple wines (Rose, 2006).

Apple cider vinegar has been used in medicine for thousands of years. It has been commonly used for a variety of conditions, including mushroom poisoning, dandruff, and toothache. During the American Civil War and World War I, it was used to treat battlefield wounds. Japanese warriors, the samurai, are thought to have drunk it to increase their strength and power. Ancient Persians drank the dilution of vinegar in apple cider to avoid the build-up of fatty tissue in the body while Romans used fire and vinegar in their Alpine conquest to break rocks. Vinegar has been used for food preservation for thousands of years and remains a valuable cleaning product today. In short, historical records indicate that apple cider vinegar from around the world is used in countless ways (Rose, 2006).

Ancient Greece

In Ancient Greece, Oxycrat was the most common beverage. water, vinegar, and honey were collected, mixed and preserved in individual vases (oxides). A remarkable physician, Hippocrates, whose doctrines ruled over Western civilization until the 18th century, (i.e., for more than 2,000 years) prescribed this mixture to treat wounds, sores, and diseases of the breath.

The Romans

The Romans drank "posca," a combination of water and vinegar that was sold on the streets in contemporary times. Posca was supposed to give you energy, while you would get drunk from wine. In Christian scriptures, it is said that the praetorian gave a sponge soaked in posca to Jesus on the cross.

It wasn't cruelty, but a symbol of the soldier's pity to a man on the cross. Acetabulum, a glass bowl used for serving vinegar, was always present at Roman banquets. Feasters would dip small pieces of bread into the vinegar and eat it throughout the meal to aid digestion.

Vinegar was contained in nearly all the recipes prepared by Apicius, a well-known Epicurean gastronomer in Roman times. Later, Columella, a Roman agricultural writer, left a few vinegar recipes; acid yeast has been used to favor fermentation, while incandescent bars and hot fir cones have been placed in wine to purify them.

The Romans had several vinegar sauces, ranging from very basic to the popular garum, which was the strange mix of ingredients to be combined with vinegar. The Romans invented the method of marinating fried fish. In his Naturalism History, Pliny the Elder recommends vinegar to treat various conditions and to make life more pleasant.

Vinegar was always available for Roman legionaries. Their daily meal before the battle was momentum, a salad made of garlic, onion, rue, goat milk, and coriander, coated with oil and vinegar.

Throughout military campaigns, vinegar was also used to quench thirst, and mixed with water, to purify the skin, to avoid and treat infections caused by camp life and small wounds.

Hannibal Barca, the famous Carthaginian general (247-183 B.C.), crossed the Alps with foot soldiers, knights, and elephants at the Piccolo San Bernardo Pass and so avoided the Roman-dominated sea during the decisive fight between Rome and Carthage. It's a famous event. It is less clear why he crossed the Alps. The paths are narrow and twisting, difficult for the massive elephants. Hannibal had huge branches between the rocks, which blocked the trail, setting them on fire. Then he had poured vinegar on hot stones, the stone was crumbly, and soldiers would smash them to get troops and animals through.

The Middle Ages and Beyond

Middle Ages

The technique for the production of vinegar improved in the Middle Ages, and Agresto was first produced using green grapes that could counterbalance condiment fat, thanks to their freshness and slight acidity.

In 1394, the newly established Vinegar Producers Association in Orléans put manufacturing technology under a code of secrecy under the penalty of expulsion by its representative. This is why the Orléans vinegar is widespread, and the business is booming. By 1580 the town and its suburbs had 33 vinegar mills as local wine, which was not very acidic or fruity, was highly suitable for the production of vinegar.

The geographic position of Orléans was also favorable: it was the last maritime port for goods coming from the west. The ships traveling along the river were very slow because of the lack of water, and by the time the wine got to the port, it was ready for vinegar processing, by correctly mixing it with the local wine.

Vinegar and the Plague

The Black Death spread all over Europe and killed one out of three people in the 14th century. Until 1670, the outbreak of the disease was marked every year at different levels.

Vinegar was believed to be great for prevention, and the people of Marseilles shielded themselves from the "fever-creating" air in 1720, the year of the last major outbreak in western Europe. They kept a vinegar-swept sponge "under the nose" without ever breathing through the mouth or swallowing saliva. Nurses supported the doctors with a vinegar basin, in which the doctors could wash their hands before the patients palpated.

When the force of the plague diminished, the walls of the homes where the sick lived were washed with vinegar.

Vinegar of the Four Thieves

In the novel 'Promessi Sposi' by Manzoni, a vinegar-treated bandage was placed around the foreheads of the Monatti- the carriers of the corpses- to avoid infections. Four of them (some people say 7) were able to sack the town scot-free during the 1720 plague outbreak in Marseille thanks to the ablutions and aromatic vinegar gargles of which the ingredients are unknown.

They were finally sentenced to death for sacking and robbery, but their lives were spared due to the vinegar they used, which became known as the Vinegar of The Four Thieves. The vinegar used in the four robberies was made by a French specialist, based on the original Marseilles recipe with many spices, cloves, and camphor and wormwood, and three pints of vinegar.

Vinegar and Cholera

A former infectious disease from remote regions of Asia, it is still prevalent in several countries in Europe and is often mistaken for acute gastroenteritis, with which it has a lot of similarities. Cholera has been treated with vinegar in any historical period. The government of Vienna passed an order almost two centuries ago (1830 and 1884), because of the cholera outbreak, that people had to wash their hands with vinegar before and after a visit to a friend or sick person, as well as fruit and vegetables before eating it. Cholera can be spread by water, so preventative action and the disinfection of food are well known.

Recent research by Franco Mecca (Franco Angeli Editore) shows that vinegar has a "simple and marked" disinfectant effect on cholera and other intestinal pathogens. In between 30 seconds-2 minutes, the vibrios on the surface of fruit and vegetables in contact with vinegar are killed.

Vinegar as a Beauty Product

Kings and princes used vinegar in the last century as a beauty product. The king of Portugal, the queen of Holland, the queen of Belgium and the princess of Wales, were selected, as the ad published in "Il Secolo" on 15 February 1873 states, to announce "that [vinegar] gives water a pleasant fragrance and has tone and soothing qualities," prevents chilblains from developing and strengthens musculature. The same ads include ammonia vinegar salt used as a disinfectant to enter hospitals, lazar houses, and "other areas where dangerous exhalations occur." Vinegar was also used for cleaning purposes in ancient and modern times. As Misette Godard points out, the situation in the European cities at the time can only be understood by comparing it with contemporary Calcutta.

Vinegar, a Multi-Purpose Product

Vinegar is a multifunctional drug; women smelled vinegar in the 19th century to restore their senses if their corset was too tight or to cure headaches. The house lady would also leave a bottle of vinegar open next to a person with influenza to prevent sickness for those who visited him/her.

Our ancestors used vinegar in the manufacture of syrups, emulsions, salts, decoctions, mouthwash, sublimates, lotions, eyewash, soap, and buffers. Vinegar has also been used for rinsing, massaging, gargling, fomenting, shaving, washing, inhaling, showering, bandaging, plastering, and many other uses.

Chapter 3:
Uses of Apple Cider Vinegar

If you're looking for information about apple cider vinegar, you've come to the right place. Acetic acid is the element that resides in vinegar and gives it its scent and taste.

It is also rumored to help with weight loss. Acetic acid helps prevent body fat and certain liver fats from building up, so it can help you achieve your targets of weight loss. Regular acetic acid intake will help you reduce the size of your abdomen and waist region.

One folk medicine used to aid people with diabetes is this vinegar. Several experiments have shown that before going to bed, drinking apple cider vinegar would give much more beneficial levels of blood sugar in the night. It also helps boost the amount of good cholesterol and lower the amount of fat in the body.

You can also use apple cider vinegar to help give relief when you suffer from dandruff. You help restore the acidic equilibrium on your scalp by mixing the vinegar with water and applying the solution to your hair. This approach is usually used for fifteen minutes at a time, only once or twice a week.

You can also use apple cider vinegar to help cure acne. This treatment is along the same lines as the cure for dandruff. Vinegar is mixed with water and dabbed into your skin's affected areas. But, be wary of this one. If the solution has too much vinegar, the vinegar will burn the body.

If you choose to use vinegar in your home remedies, you should be careful. You risk damaging your throat and teeth if you drink vinegar. You should consult your doctor before using vinegar in your diet if you have low potassium levels or osteoporosis. If you use too much, you may also damage your stomach and liver.

If you are still searching for more information about the advantages and drawbacks of using apple cider vinegar, a quick online search will help you find out more. There are plenty of resources out there to tell you what remedies you should look for and use. It's up to you!

It is sold in liquid form that is not filtered and unpasteurized. The mother of vinegar is found deposited at the base of the water in deep soil containing primarily acetic acid. Unlike others used to bake, this vinegar is used for health purposes. It is confirmed that diseases such as indigestion and pneumonia have been controlled. Several individuals have been treated by the use of apple cider vinegar combined with honey for digestive tract infections caused by bacteria.

Some also claim that they play a role in reducing body weight by burning fat through faster metabolism in combination with vitamin B6 and lecithin. This vinegar's supporters recommend taking it for burning fat and losing weight before each meal.

Some studies have shown that lowering blood glucose levels can help people with diabetes.

Health Benefits

Proponents argue that apple cider vinegar (and vinegar in general) can improve your health in a variety of ways. A few of these claims are supported by science. Here's a glance forward.

Blood Sugar Level

The acetic acid in vinegar appears to obstruct enzymes that help absorb starch, leading to a smaller sized reaction of blood glucose after starchy meals like pasta or bread.

Scientists examined previously published medical research studies on the effects of vinegar intake with a meal in a report released in 2017 and discovered that vinegar assisted in reducing blood sugar and insulin levels after a meal.

Attempt adding a splash to salads, vinaigrettes, sauces, and marinades to integrate apple cider vinegar into your meals. If you have prediabetes or diabetes, make sure to talk to your doctor if you are thinking about using more substantial quantities that are generally used in baking.

Vinegar can interfere with treatment for diabetes, and people with certain forms of nutritional conditions, such as gastroparesis, should not use it.

Weight Loss

Proponents claim that it may have a satiating effect to drink vinegar before or with a meal. A Japanese study investigated the effects of daily intake of vinegar on body fat in obese adults. After the 12-week experiment, people who had eaten vinegar had a tiny decrease in body weight from one to two pounds. There was also a decrease in body mass index (BMI), waist circumference, triglycerides, and visceral fat.

Nonetheless, to understand the link between vinegar and weight, further studies are needed. When used for weight loss purposes, people tend to consume more than average amounts of apple cider vinegar, some even taking it in tablet form. Nevertheless, there is a possibility that drugs may damage the digestive tract.

From avocado facials to honey scrubs, hitting the kitchen cabinet in the hope of getting cleaner, smoother skin is nothing new. But is apple cider vinegar (ACV), another superfood ingredient, worthy of a spot on your vanity in the bathroom?

It's not surprising if you've considered using this staple pantry item to help treat acne or other skin conditions like eczema, psoriasis, or rosacea. Due to its reputation for healing common infections and wounds or lowering blood sugar in people with type 2 diabetes, ACV's popularity has only increased in recent years, as some research shows.

Researchers have mixed views on the use of ACV as a skin condition treatment. Anecdotally, both successes and adverse reactions have been heard. If you have a mild condition, it may help, but it's probably not going to be the be-all-end-all for more severe cases.

The outer layer of your body, the epidermis, is like a brick wall. Water comes out when you break it apart, and irritants can come in. Many facial washes, toners, and bar soaps are just too hard and strip that layer. Skin's pH is slightly acidic, and so is ACV, so if you have dry skin, you can usually use it without removing the epidermis. You want to keep the lipid layer in place to keep the irritants from penetrating the skin.

Acne

Acne forms a plug (a blackhead or a whitehead) when keratin, the main protein in your skin, builds up in a pore. Unlike citric acid, AHAs remove the keratin to open and drain the pore, helping to make pores appear smaller and to improve the appearance of acne. Retinoids and benzoyl peroxide have achieved the same effect.

We know that breaking down keratin can help with acne, and ACV contains AHAs, so there is potential, but there are simply not functional studies to prove that.

If you are already using an anti-acne rinse or acne cream, and the treatment appears to irritate the body, causing dryness and peeling, and if you add ACV to your regimen, you may be removing the epidermis.

The object is accomplished by letting out all the moisture and everything inside— air pollutants, irritants, bacteria — in. Everyone is a bit different, and oily skin is likely to have a higher tolerance to apply more acidic products. There is a much lower threshold for sensitive, dry skin. There's no one-size-fits-all recommendation. Using ACV is less risky for teens with oily skin and acne because their skin is more resistant to irritation. The oil protects the skin's outer layer, and in a younger person, it comes back faster than an older adult with drier skin. Hair Benefits: In the medicine cabinet as well as in the kitchen cupboard, you may want to start stashing apple cider vinegar. This favorite ingredient can do more than just dress salads and make pickles — it's also a great all-in-one beauty product on a budget for you.

Apple cider vinegar can help you look beautiful from head to toe when used in your makeup routine. Hard soaps and shampoos often strip hair and skin of their natural oils, allowing you to feel dry all over. Apple cider vinegar acidity counteracts this cycle and in turn, improves the typical pH values of your skin and hair.

Make sure you get the right things. For the most beauty benefits, choose an organic brand of raw apple cider vinegar. Here are some useful tips on how to use apple cider vinegar to make your hair and skin look good.

For Hair

Apple cider vinegar removes product buildup, clumpy residue, and gunk from hair. Apple cider vinegar will revitalize your hair's body, making it moist and shiny when used daily in your natural hair care routine. The vinegar also acts by removing the skin cuticula, making it reflect light from it. In other words, this makes your hair super shiny!

Over the past few years, makeup advocates and medical experts have praised apple cider vinegar for its many health benefits, with many drinking apple cider vinegar to help clear their skin or even lose weight as part of their beauty routine. Like anything else, ACV may not be a miracle cure for any health-related issues, but helping you get bright, healthy hair can be an easy, economical workaround,

whether you buy products such as apple cider vinegar shampoo or whipping a DIY hair rinse at home using ACV.

Chapter 4:
Apple Cider for Moisturizing, Rejuvenating and Exfoliating your Skin

The thought of putting a smelly, sour liquid like apple cider on your face may put you off, but if you learn and believe in its benefits, you will gladly use it regularly. Although there many great-smelling, better advertised facial cleansers available in the market, ACV still gets the vote of naturalists. This is because it is made from naturally fermented apples and it does not contain any preservatives or toxins that can be harmful to your health in the long run. Just make sure to use the raw, unfiltered one that still contains the "mother".

It also contains alpha-hydroxy acids that gets rid of dead cells and help reveal your healthier, younger-looking skin underneath. Unlike its commercial counterparts, the alpha hydroxy acids in ACV are naturally occurring and are not added into it.

If you start noticing age spots on your skin, simply apply undiluted ACV directly on the affected area using a cotton ball. Leave on for about 20 to 30 minutes and rinse off with cool water. Apply regularly for 2 months and you will start seeing significant improvements in your skin.

<u>To help improve your skin, try these recipes:</u>

For Smoother Skin

8 oz. apple cider vinegar

Warm bath water

If you have a bath tub, fill your tub with warm water and mix in vinegar. Soak in it for 15 to 20 minutes. If you don't have a tub, fill a basin or a pail with warm water and mix in the vinegar. Slowly wet your entire body with the bath water using a dipper.

Apple cider is alkaline and its pH level is the same with the pH level of your skin's mantle layer that is why it can effectively restore balance and make your skin smoother and softer.

Skin Toner

1 tablespoonapple cider vinegar

2 cups water

Mix them together in a glass bottle or container. Moisten a cotton ball with the mixture and wipe on your entire face and neck. Leave it to dry and allow the smell to go away. Do not rinse. The alpha hydroxy acids in ACV stimulate circulation while acetic acid helps minimize pores.

Acne Remover

1 cup apple cider vinegar

3 cups rooibos tea

1 droptea tree essential oil

1 droporegano essential oil

Prepare 3 cups of hot water and let the rooibos tea soak for 10 to 15 minutes. When tea is cool enough, add ACV and essential oils. Mix thoroughly. Transfer in a glass container or PET bottle with tight lid. Shake container before every use. Soak cotton balls with mixture and apply gently on acne areas. Allow to dry and do not rinse.

Do this procedure regularly before going to bed at night and an hour before you take your shower in the morning. This mixture is also great for oily skin as it helps balance its pH level and prevent overproduction of oil.

Sunburn Relief

1/2 cup apple cider vinegar

4 cupswater

Douse a clean washcloth with the solution and apply on affected skin. The acidity of ACV restores balance on your skin. It also prevents blisters and supports faster healing.

For Rejuvenated and Moisturized Skin

1 cup apple cider vinegar

3 cups green tea

1 drop tea tree essential oil

Soak green tea in 3 cups of hot water for 15 minutes. When cool enough, transfer in a glass bottle or container with tight cover. Add essential oil and ACV. Shake well to mix thoroughly. If the smell is too much for you, apply mixture to your skin in the evening before you sleep. Your skin will feel and look fresher and younger the next day.

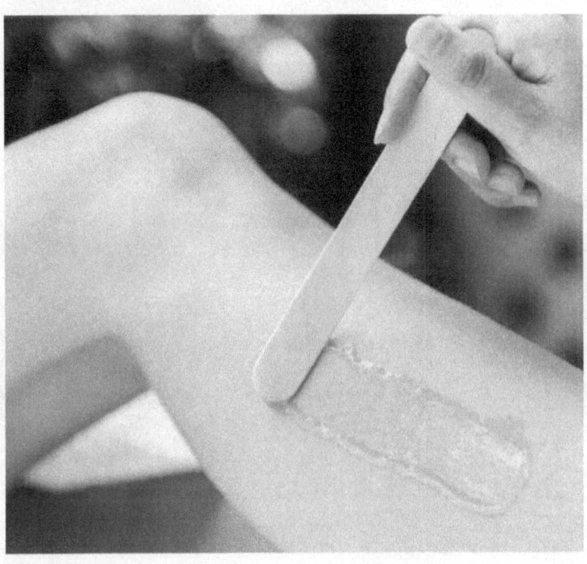

Skin Perfecting Mask

1 teaspoon rose water

1 teaspoon deep sea mud

1/4 teaspoon apple cider vinegar

1/8 teaspoon yogurt

1 teaspoon kombucha

1/16 teaspoon nutritional yeast

Note: You can use arrowroot powder as substitute for deep sea mud, and plain water for rose water. If you want the mask to be thicker, add more deep sea mud or yogurt. If you want it thinner, add more rose water.

Mix all ingredients together in a small bowl. Apply evenly on your face and leave overnight. You will have clearer, softer, glowing skin the day after.

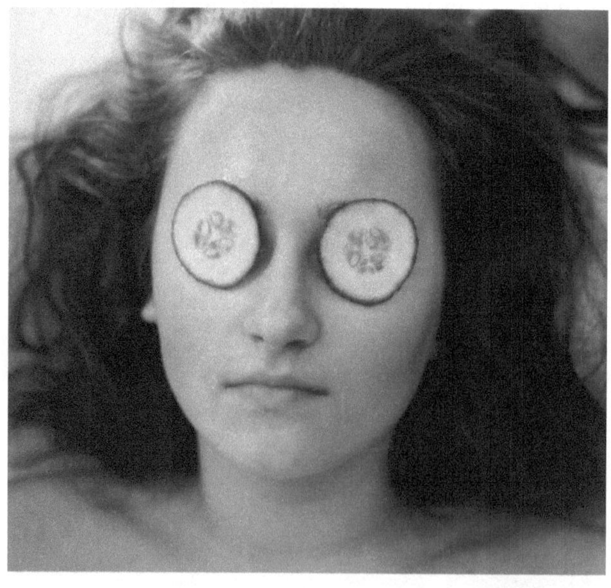

Razor Bump Remedy

1 tablespoonapple cider vinegar

Cotton balls

Moisten cotton ball with undiluted ACV and wipe on the affected area. Leave on for 5 minutes and rinse with cold water. Apple cider has anti-inflammatory properties that can relieve irritated skin. The acetic acid in it softens the skin and promotes hair growth.

Bruise Remedy

1 teaspoon apple cider vinegar

Cotton pad

Moisten cotton pad with undiluted apple cider vinegar. Secure it on the bruise with a bandage. Let it stay for an hour before removing. The anti-inflammatory properties of ACV can relieve injured skin and its acetic acid can promote healing and increase blood circulation to the affected area.

Treatment for Bug Bite

1 teaspoon apple cider vinegar

Cotton ball

Apply ACV on the bug bite using the cotton ball. This will provide instant relief. The anti-inflammatory properties of the vinegar can reduce swelling and its alpha hydroxy acids reduce itching. Its natural acidity also supports faster healing.

Apple cider vinegar contains beta carotene that helps repair damage due to free radicals. The result is a healthier and younger complexion. It also has antibacterial and antiseptic properties that protect your skin from pollution and bacteria. Also, apple cider has a pH level of 4.5 to 5.5, which is close to the ideal pH level of the skin, making it effective in restoring your pH balance. This is how ACV keeps your skin healthy, fresh and young.

Chapter 5:
Apple Cider for Shiny, Healthy Hair

Apple cider vinegar is a by-product of fermenting apples. Apples are rich in potassium, calcium, pectin and malic acid that are fortified further with enzymes and good bacteria after the fermentation. Raw, unfiltered ACV keeps all the nutrients intact, making it better than the filtered version.

For healthier, softer, shinier and more luscious locks, try out the following hair rinse recipes:

For Dry Hair

2 to 4 tablespoons apple cider vinegar

16 oz. water

1 dropmyrrh essential oil

Note: If you are a beginner, use a lesser amount of ACV and gradually increase after a few times of use.

Mix the ingredients thoroughly in a small bowl. After shampooing and rinsing your hair, dry with towel. Apply mixture to your damp hair, making sure to cover your entire scalp and massage through your hair. Leave on for 2 minutes. Rinse thoroughly with cold water.

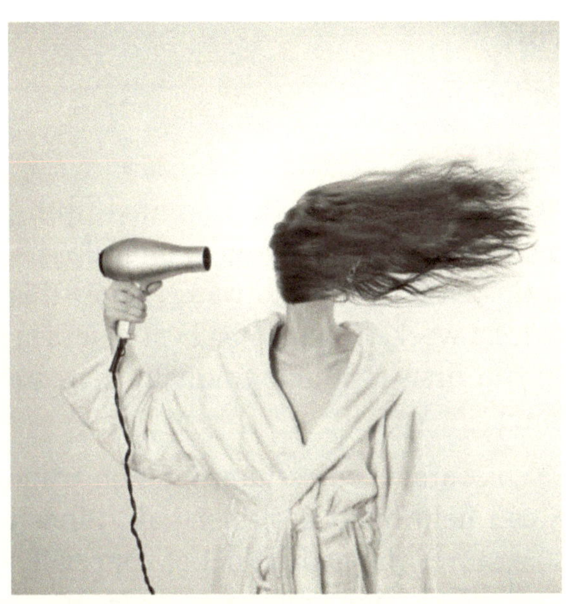

To Remove Residue Build Up

1/4 cup apple cider vinegar

2 cups water

Mix ingredients and apply on hair after shampooing. Rinse with cold water.

For Oily Hair

4 teaspoons apple cider vinegar

16 oz. water

1 drop lavender oil

Apply mixture on hair after shampooing. Leave on for 5 minutes. Rinse with cold water.

For Dandruff

1 cup apple cider vinegar

3 cupswarm water

Mix together in a container with a pointed tip to ensure that you can apply the liquid directly on your scalp. Leave on for 5 minutes and rinse it off with cold water. Apply this mixture no more than twice a week. It would be best to lessen the amount of ACV when you first try it and gradually increase its amount as you go along.

Apple cider also contains potassium, Vitamin B and Vitamin C, all of which can help build healthier hair. Since it is slightly acidic, it also restores the natural pH of your hair, which leads to shinier, smoother, and tangle-free hair. It also has anti-fungal, antibacterial and antiviral properties that bring relief to dandruff and flaky scalp.

Chapter 6:
Apple Cider for Detox and Losing Weight

This wonder vinegar has long been used by naturalists and herbalist to purge unwanted toxins in the body. Aside from improving your hair and skin, it also helps boost your immunity and lose weight. The cleansing properties of apple cider help your body get rid of accumulated waste, therefore, giving you more energy and enhancing your immunity.

Apple cider detoxifies your body by improving your bowel movement so you can flush out wastes effectively. It also purifies your blood and enhances circulation through its powerful enzymes that break down bad cholesterol to prevent them from clogging your arteries.

This vinegar also helps maintain a healthy alkaline level in your body to prevent inflammation. In addition, it also breaks down mucus, which helps cleanse the lymph nodes. This boosts lymph circulation, which leads to a healthier immune system.

Here are ACV recipes for Detox:

Basic Cider Drink

2 tablespoons apple cider vinegar

1 teaspoon honey

1 cup warm water

Mix in a tall glass and drink in the morning in an empty stomach. This drink is very easy to prepare. Aside from detoxifying your body, it also gives you more energy and helps keep you awake in the morning.

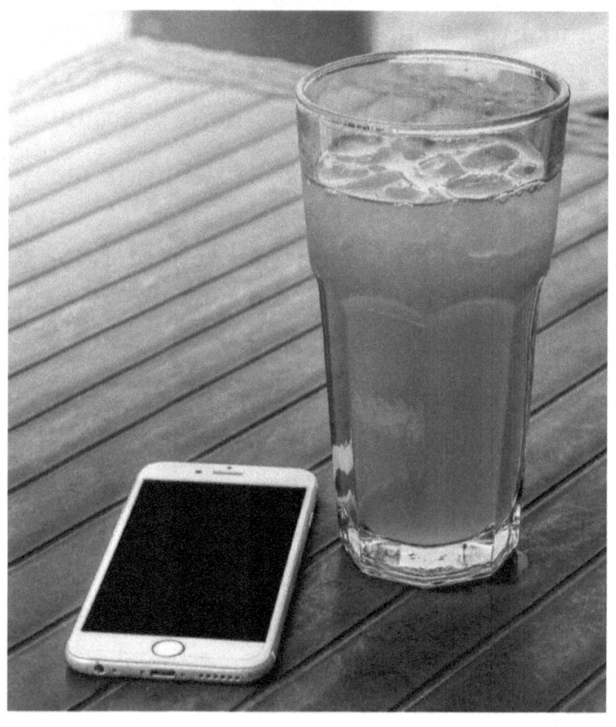

Lemon Cider Drink

12 ounces drinking water

4 tablespoons apple cider vinegar

1 teaspoon cinnamon, ground

1 lemon

1 pinch cayenne pepper

4 tablespoons honey, raw

Mix all ingredients in a tall glass. You can add 5 to 6 ice cubes if you want it cold. This drink helps boost your metabolism and aids in detoxification and weight loss.

Apple Cider Cranberry Detox

1/4 cup cranberry juice, unsweetened

1 tablespoonapple cider vinegar

1 tablespoon lemon juice

1 cup water

2 tablespoons honey

Add all ingredients in a tall glass and mix. You can add ice cubes if you prefer cold drinks. This concoction is great in cleansing the kidneys, lymphatic system, digestive system and liver, which all helps in removing wastes and toxins out of your body.

Apple Cider Detox Bath

4 ounces apple cider vinegar

2 cups baking soda

2 cups Epsom salt

Fill your bathtub with warm water. Mix the rest of the ingredients into the tub and soak in it for 30 minutes or until the water in your tub gets cold. Pat yourself dry. Do not rinse. It is best to do this at night before you go to sleep as it also relaxes your entire body so you can have better sleep. The baking soda helps remove excess oil and exfoliate your skin while the Epsom salt helps pull out toxins from your body.

Weight Loss Drink

1 cup warm water

30ml apple cider vinegar

Mix together and drink before every meal. This drink will make you feel full longer and aids in lowering your insulin and glucose levels.

ACV Tea

1 cup boiling water

3 teaspoons apple cider vinegar

1 tablespoon honey (optional)

1 pouch/bag green tea

Let the green tea steep in boiling water for 10 to 15 minutes. Mix in honey and apple cider vinegar when the tea is cool enough. Do not add vinegar in hot water as it can destroy the healthy enzymes in it. You can prepare this in advance and double the recipe so you can bring it with you anywhere. It detoxifies your body and help break down excess fats.

Apple Cider Immunity Booster

1 teaspoon apple cider vinegar

1 cup green tea

1 lemon, juiced

1 teaspoon honey

1 inch ginger

1 pinch cinnamon

Steep green tea and ginger in boiling water for 10 to 15 minutes or until water is cool. Mix in the rest of the ingredients. This drink helps boost your immunity for better detox results. It is also anti-inflammatory and gives you the kick start you need in the morning.

Garlic Honey Cider Drink

2 teaspoons apple cider vinegar

2 teaspoons honey

1 clove garlic, crushed

1 pinch cayenne pepper

1/4 fruit lemon, juiced

Mix all ingredients in a tall glass and add cold water. Drink this mixture before every meal. It reduces your cravings for food, enhances your immune system and boosts your metabolism.

The organic enzymes and acids found in cider vinegar increase your metabolism, which results to faster fat burning. This translates to weight loss. It also curbs your cravings for food, therefore, you eat less and you feel and look slimmer. Also, it has high potassium and fiber that help lower your blood sugar. It also hydrates your body and prevents water retention.

Apple cider is a natural way to detoxify and lose weight. Plus, it is much cheaper in comparison to supplements and it does not have harmful side effects that only show after some time.

Chapter 12 - How to Make your Own Apple Cider Vinegar at Home

If you are the type of person who wants to do everything on your own, this is good news. You can prepare apple cider vinegar on your own home. It's easy and way cheaper in comparison to market-bought ones.

What you need:

10 organic apples

Water

Cheesecloth

1 glass jar with wide mouth

How to do it:

1. Wash the apples thoroughly and allow them to dry.

2. Cut the apples into cubes. Include the peels and cores, but remove the stem.

3. Transfer the apple cubes into the glass jar and fill with water. Make sure to cover all the apples with water.

4. Cover the jar with cheesecloth and secure with a rubber band. Keep it in a warm, dark place for about 2 to 3 weeks. You will start to notice scum on top of the liquid.

5. Strain the liquid and transfer back into the same glass container. Cover with cheesecloth secured with a rubber band. Put it back into the same dark, warm area for another 4 to 6 weeks. Remember to stir the liquid every 2 to 3 days.

6. At week 4, taste the liquid if it is sour enough for you. If not, continue fermenting until your desired sourness is achieved.

7. Transfer in a glass bottle and enjoy it as you would.

Making your own apple cider vinegar is so easy. It does not require any special skills. It does require some patience since you have to wait for a few months before you can finally enjoy its benefits. Nonetheless, if you don't want to wait that long, you can always buy in the market. Just make sure to choose the one that still contains the mother to enjoy its optimum benefits.

Tips:

Make sure to use sterilized glass jar for fermenting and storing. Prior to fermenting, make sure that there are no soap residues or debris left in the bottle as it will affect the quality and taste of your ACV. Your cheesecloth should also be clean and dry. Remember, when the scum that forms on top of your mixture is white, then that means that it's good. However, if it is of different color other than white (black, blue, green or gray), then you have to discard it. This means bad bacteria has infested your ferment and it can be harmful to your health if you consume it.

If you have leftover apple peels and core, do not throw them. You can ferment them instead and turn them into apple cider. If possible, use organic apples to minimize your risk of ingesting pesticides used in commercially grown apples.

Chapter 7:
Other BIG Benefits of Apple Cider Vinegar

Aside from all the benefits mentioned above, apple cider still has a lot more to offer.

Natural preservative – The acetic acid in ACV kills pathogens and bacteria such as E. coli that causes food to spoil. The shelf-life of meat dishes can be extended by adding some of the vinegar into them. Since the ancient times, it has already been used as a natural disinfectant and preservative

Lowers blood sugar levels – Studies show that taking 2 tablespoons of ACV prior to eating reduces blood sugar by 34%. It can also improve insulin sensitivity by 19% to 34%. Numerous studies show that taking it before meals significantly reduces blood sugar responses during meal and increases insulin sensitivity, but this does not mean you can go overboard with your carb intake especially if you are diabetic.

Natural massage treatment – When you have sore or painful hands and feet, massage directly with undiluted ACV and you will find relief and enjoy the benefits of conventional massage.

Natural flea repellent for pets – If your pet is infested with fleas, just mix one part apple cider to one part water and spray generously on your pet's fur. Massage until all the fur are coated. Rinse well with water. Repeat procedure every day for 1 to two weeks or until all fleas are gone.

Natural bathroom deodorizer – To keep your bathroom or any room smelling fresh, use apple cider vinegar. For your bathroom, pour some of it into your toilet and leave it overnight. Rinse with water the next day. It will leave your bathroom smelling like apples.

Natural home cleaner – To keep your house clean, dilute 1/2 cup ACV to 1 cup water and use to clean your mirrors, windows, tabletops, countertops, kitchen surfaces, oven, microwave and many more.

Natural candida cure – Apple cider is loaded with good enzymes that help relieve Candida. It is a fungus (form of yeast) that is normally found in the body, but in very small amounts. They are usually found in the intestine and in the mouth. When they thrive and multiply in abnormal proportions, thrush and other undesirable conditions may develop. Taking apple cider vinegar every day cures Candida and its symptoms.

Heartburn relief – Taking one teaspoon of apple cider followed by a cup of water can help relieve heartburn. Research suggests that the acidity of ACV neutralizes the stomach acid, reducing heartburn. **This treatment does not work if you have ulcer.**

Athletes foot relief – Mix one cup ACV to 4 cups lukewarm (not warm) water in a tall basin and soak your feet for 15 to 20 minutes. The antibacterial and antifungal properties of this vinegar kill the fungus that causes odor to your feet. Do this once a day preferably before going to bed.

Upset stomach soother – If you feel bloated, gassy and constipated or if you suspect food poisoning, mix 2 tablespoons ACV to 1 cup water and drink. In case of food poisoning, you still need to see a doctor after drinking ACV.

Baking aid – It turns out that vinegar can help give batters a lift, making them more moist and spongy. Since ACV has a mild taste, it is almost undetectable, making it a favorite among chefs and bakers.

Sore throat relief – If you feel like your throat is starting to itch and ache or if you already have symptoms of sore throat, then start mixing up 1/4 cup cider vinegar to 1 cup warm water and use it to gargle. The acidity of this vinegar soothes the throat and prevents the bacteria from propagating.

Natural relief for cough and colds – The antibacterial properties of ACV help ward off cough and colds. Also, its potassium content loosens the mucus in your sinuses, allowing you to breathe better. Mix 2 tablespoons of apple cider to 1 cup warm water and 1 teaspoon honey. Drink it as needed.

Chapter 8:
What is the 8:16 Intermittent Fasting Diet?

Anyone can follow the 8:16 intermittent fasting diet. If done properly, those who tried it out can achieve amazing results not only in their physique, but also in their overall health and fitness.

The 8:16 IF diet is fundamentally a diet protocol where you have breakfast later than usual and eat dinner in the early evening. This eating schedule promotes losing excess body fat and better control over blood sugar levels.

The 8:16 term refers to eating within an 8-hour period and fasting for the rest of the 16 hours in a day. All the calories you need in a day will be consumed within this short eating period.

The IF diet is actually more of a lifestyle rather than a diet. The idea is that fasting periods will encourage the body to use fats for energy. This is shifting the body's energy source from the calories from immediate food intake to stored fats.

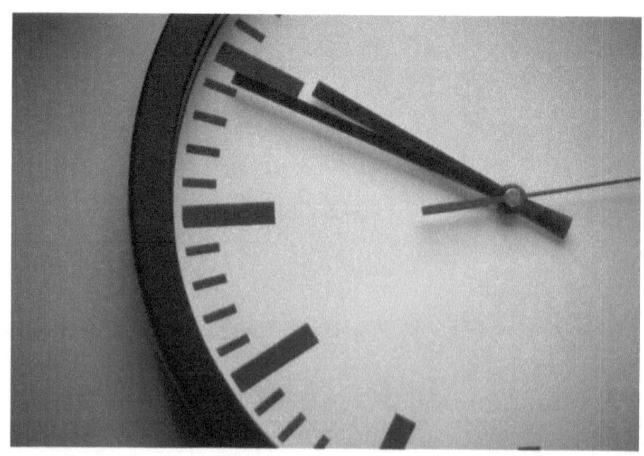

Basic 8:16 protocol

The thing is that you will sleep off about 4 to 8 hours of the 16-hour fasting period. You can spend the remaining hours focusing on other activities, like your work, hobby and workout.

You generally start fasting after your early dinner. Typically, you will be spending around 3 hours or so doing your pre-bed activities, like catching up on work, wrapping up your day with some leisure activities (e.g., reading, surfing the net, watching TV, doing some light household chores, preparing next day's presentations or stuff you need, cleaning up, tidying up, etc.) or doing some light workout.

In this diet, you will be eating breakfast later in the day. Instead of eating breakfast between 6AM and 8AM, you can eat around 11AM.

Think of it this way, you get to have more time in the morning to get more things done. You won't be rushing in the morning to prepare breakfast. You free up some time to do other things like going through your materials to check everything is ready for your day's lineup of activities. You can finally get that morning run you wanted to do for the longest time. You may even squeeze in a few moments of yoga or other light workout to start your day.

What Intermittent Fasting does IN the body

When you fast, you trigger some amazing processes in the body that are otherwise inactive or not happening at full force. For example, during fasting periods, apophagy is accelerated. This refers to a process, which involves eating dead and old, worn out cells. This process is important because it is the body's way of cleaning out dead, old, damaged and useless cells. These are brought out from within the tissues and excreted. This process works in clearing out the tissues of potentially harmful buildup of non-functional cells, along with toxins.

When you work out during fasting periods (yes, it is possible), you get to see greater results from your workout routine. Working out while you are fasting optimizes favorable hormonal processes you got going whenever you fast. Several hormones are either activated or inhibited, all of which can contribute to greater responsiveness of the muscle tissues.

During fasting periods, the muscles are more responsive to the presence of insulin. When you work out during this time, you can trigger greater anabolic response. This will help you get buffed faster. You build lean muscles while you also develop endurance and better muscle performance.

This IF diet is ideal for people who are planning to lose weight AND build lean muscles. This diet also works perfectly for those who wish to burn fats for sustained weight loss and keep fat accumulation at a minimum.

Other processes stimulated by this diet include:

- Increased flow of blood to the fat cells

- Slight increase in metabolic rate

- Reduced insulin levels

- Release of fatty acids that can be used as more sustainable energy for the cells

- Increase in the concentrations of norepinephrine and epinephrine

Chapter 9:
Basics of the 8:16 I.F. Diet

It is pretty simple - eat within 8 hours and fast for the next 16 hours. You do this every day without any cheat days. Why do you need cheat days if you already have an 8-hour window each day to eat whatever you want? Remember, IF is not about eating special foods. It is more on giving your body time to burn fats for energy by fasting.

A 16-hour fast can be quite challenging, especially if you are used to eating all day long. A few discomforts may be experienced such as:

- Irritability

- Restlessness

- Cravings

- Crankiness

- Inability to focus

- Slight weakness

- Nagging hunger

These discomforts will eventually go away as the body turns to burning fats for energy. Drinking a lot of water during the fasting state can help reduce these discomforts.

If the 16-hour fast becomes exceptionally difficult, then you can opt to perform the 8:16 intermittent fast slowly. Instead of going cold turkey and fast immediately, you can train your body to adjust to a new eating schedule.

Our body is a trainable machine. When we eat at specific times each day, our body learns to anticipate it. For example, we usually eat lunch at 12 noon. Our body learns and adapts to this schedule. By 11:30 AM, we start to feel hungry. Our stomach acids increase in anticipation of food we will soon be eating. Our minds start to wander towards thoughts of food, too. If we can train our bodies to eat regularly, we can also train it to wait a little longer before feeling hungry. It is possible and numerous people are already successful at this.

To train your body to endure a 16-hour fast, you can start with small steps. Today, extend your breakfast time by an hour or eat dinner a little earlier. For instance, your usual breakfast time is at 6AM. Today, make it 7AM. Tomorrow, make it at 8AM and so on until you finally get to skip it altogether. With dinner, eat earlier each day. For example, you are used to eating dinner at 9PM. Tonight, eat earlier, like at 8PM. Keep adjusting until you have compressed your overall eating period in a day to 8 hours.

A lot of people find doing it slowly more effective and easier. The discomforts during the adjustment period are less intense than when doing the 8:16 cold turkey style. The key is to try a method and adjust according to how your body reacts to the new schedule you are implementing.

How the 8:16 IF diet works

Fast for 16 hours and eat only within 8 hours. Most people will think that this will cause them to experience extreme hunger. Normally, we eat all day - from the time we get up in the morning and until we finally go to sleep at night. That will be averaging anywhere from 12 to 14 hours. This is called the fed state.

In this state, the body focuses more on digesting and absorbing recently eaten foods. These processes can take up to several hours. During the fed state, the body's fat burning processes are at a minimum. It is hard for the body to burn stored fats during the fed state because it relies on the energy derived from recent food consumption.

Insulin levels are high during the fed state. This is a response to the influx of glucose from foods. This higher insulin level also hinders fat burning.

After the fed state, the body enters the post-absorptive state. In this state, the body is neither digesting nor processing food. This usually lasts for about 1 to 2 hours after you last ate a meal.

After the post-absorptive state, if you still haven't eaten or drank anything that contains calories, your body enters the fasted state.

During the fasting period, your digestive system does not actively digest solid foods. Instead, it concentrates on fully metabolizing and absorbing the nutrients from foods. This becomes an opportunity to utilize foods fully and turn these into readily usable energy. This energy is easily used up by the body. Efficient energy use lessens the possibility of converting excess calories into fats.

In the fasted state, levels of insulin are low. The inhibitory effect of insulin on fat burning is reduced; hence, the body can turn on its fat burning processes at full force. This is why people who go on intermittent fasts burn fats and lose weight without changing their current diet. Even if they still eat the same kinds of foods every day, weight loss is evident.

Steady weight loss is achievable in the 8:16 intermittent fasting diet. This is because the cells burn glycogen stores for energy during the fasted state. When you eat again to break the fast, your body will turn energy into glycogen, instead of turning it into fat cells. This further enhances weight maintenance by reducing the amount of food that gets turned and stored as fats.

Chapter 10:
Preparing for the 8:16 IF Diet

Proper preparation is crucial if you want the entire fasting process to be a little bit easier to do and get the best results.

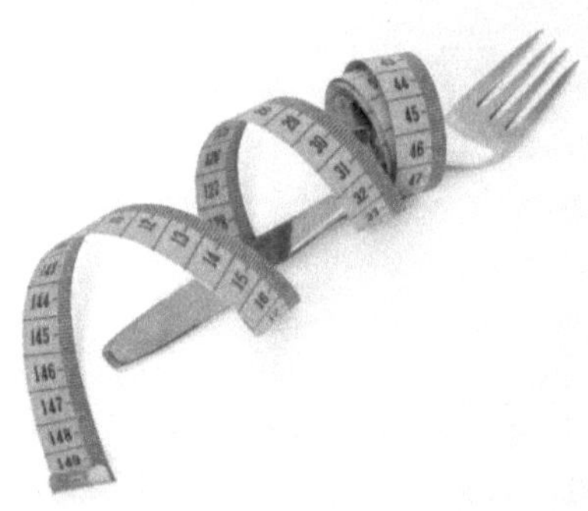

You can't haphazardly set a fasting schedule and eat indiscriminately during the eating window. If you want to beef up and not suffer through the fasting periods, you have to achieve energy balance. That will require a little math.

#1: Determine your goal

Why are you going for the 8:16 Diet? Is it only to lose weight? Is it to maintain current weight? Is it to build muscles, lose weight and keep losing weight? Set your goals first. Everything depends on your set goal.

For example, you want to lose fat. Your primary goal as of now is to lose excess fat, which gives you bulges in the wrong places.

#2: Assess your activity level

After setting down the goal, you need to determine the number of calories you need in a day to achieve this goal. Check your goal against this simple table to determine your body weight multiplier.

Get an honest assessment of the level of your daily activities. It should correspond to your current activity level - not with the activity level you plan to have to lose weight. If your activity level is sedentary, then compute based on that level even if you plan to start jogging next week.

How active are you? Do you spend long hours in a chair, such as doing computer work or a desk job? Are you on your feet all day, but do not do additional exercises? Do you jog every day or hit the gym?

Your activity level is an estimate of the number of calories your body uses up each day.

Description	Body weight multiplier (cal/lb)
Sedentary	10-11
Lightly active	11-12
Moderately active	12-13
Very active	14-15
Extremely active	18-19

#3: Calculating for calories needed to achieve goal

For example, you are 250 pounds and your main goal is to lose weight. Check your current lifestyle at the table above. Let's say you are lightly active.

You have 2 main ways to calculate your weight loss calorie intake. One, you can take your current weight and multiply it with your current activity level. In this instance:

11 x 250 lbs. = 2, 750

12 x 250 lbs. = 3, 000

That means your daily calorie count should be between 2, 750 to 3, 000 per day. You follow this calorie intake for about 2 weeks and see how your body reacts to it. Are you losing weight? The idea behind this method is the assumption that you are eating more than what your body can burn. By setting it to within this range, you are only eating what your body can burn.

Weight loss can happen by burning stored fats to keep your organs working and for homeostasis. Then again, you need to monitor your weight and observe how your body responds. This method comes with a risk that you only maintain your current weight. You will only notice minimal weight loss.

The second method is to choose your target weight and multiply it by the body weight multiplier. For example, your current weight is 250 pound and you want it to go down to 180 pounds. To set your daily calorie intake for that goal:

11 x 180 lbs. = 1, 980

12 x 180 lbs. = 2, 160

This computation gives you a daily calorie intake of between 1, 980 and 2, 160 to reduce your current weight level to 180 pounds. As with the first method, observe how your body reacts to this calorie range. Try to start at the middle range or the lower one if you think you can. If you notice you are losing too much weight or too fast, you can increase towards the upper range (2, 160 calories per day). If you think you are not losing enough weight, you can reduce to the lower limit (1, 980 calories).

#4: Calculating macros

Your macros refer to the ratios of the macronutrients in your diet. These are the proteins, fats and carbohydrates. You also include the calories in your macros computations. Getting the correct macros ratios is important if you want to use 8:16 intermittent fasting diet for continued fat loss.

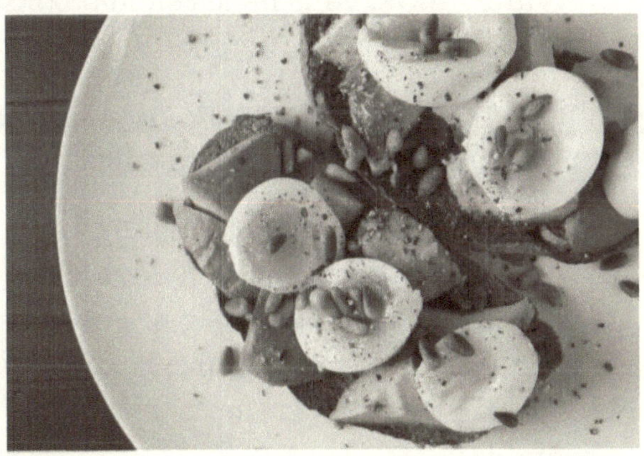

But I thought I can eat anything and everything during the eating window?

Yes, that does not change. This recommendation on the macros ratio is meant to promote steady weight loss. Sure, you will lose weight on the 8:16 even if you still eat pizza, burgers, steaks and fried foods. Even if you still enjoy luscious desserts and rich snacks, you will still lose weight as long as you follow the 16-hour fast, 8-hour eating window.

If you want to make the most out of your 16-hour fast, then have your macros correct.

The macros ratio recommended by the 8:16 IF diet is as follows:

- On non-training days, calorie intake should be 30% below maintenance level. For example, you have calculated your daily calorie intake at 1, 980. On days you are not training, your calorie intake is recommended to be at 1, 386.

- On training days, your calorie intake should be at maintenance levels. In the same example as above, your intake should be 1, 980.

- On training days, your meals should consist more of carbohydrates and less of fats.

- On non-training days, meals should have higher fat contents and lower in carbohydrates.

- On all days, regardless if training or non-training days, protein intake should be high. It should be 1.5 grams per pound of bodyweight. For example, if you weigh 250 pounds, protein intake on all days should be: 250 pounds x 1.5 grams per pound = 375 grams of proteins.

Proteins are critical in building lean muscles. Fats and calories work as energy sources. When you train, you burn carbohydrates better. That means less gets to be converted into fats and stored in the tissues. On non-training days, your main energy source should be fats.

Chapter 11:
What to Eat While Intermittent Fasting

Sure, the term "intermittent fasting" or "fasting" means not eating. However, this diet is not about starving yourself. It is also not about obsessively counting each calorie present in your food and drinks. This is not a CRaP (calorie restriction as primary) type of diet. IF firmly believes that starving yourself is setting yourself up for failure. You won't get healthy if you starve yourself. You won't beef up if you do not feed your muscles. You will definitely not experience steady weight loss if you starve yourself.

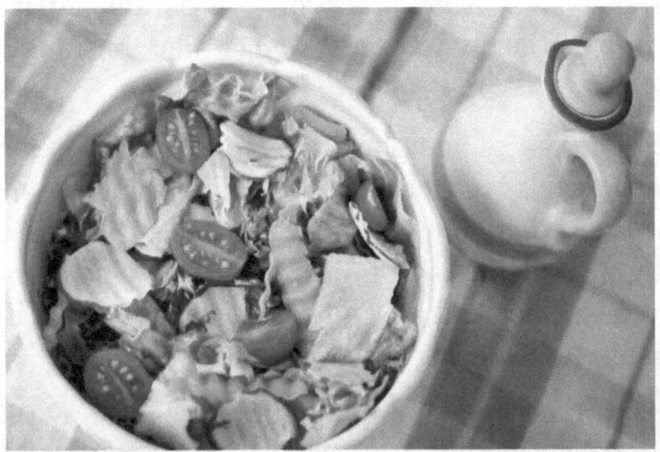

Intermittent fasting is giving your body the right amount of calories it needs to perform its many functions. Then why does it include fasting? What will fasting aim to achieve?

Imagine your body as a paper shredder. Eating is like feeding the shredder with a bunch of papers. Fasting is similar to pausing from inserting (feeding) paper to the shredder. This pause allows the machine to process what you just fed it.

Try cramming batches of paper nonstop to the paper shredder. Soon, you will have problems such as jamming.

This same thing happens in the body. If you keep feeding, it will put its efforts into digesting and storing food with the intention of dealing with it later. The body has the natural inclination to work on food it has at hand, store it for later burning when all the food has been digested. If you keep on eating, the body can't actually convert and use energy.

Research has actually demonstrated that eating small meals frequently is not going to help you with weight loss. It won't have a lasting positive effect on your metabolism either. Constant eating is not going to give your body time to process food completely. It will constantly trigger the system to break down foods with little time for doing anything else. You have to let your body rest from processing foods and let it turn its attention to other important things like burning fat and building muscles.

Research has also demonstrated that eating large and infrequent meals is better than eating smaller and more frequent meals. Larger and less frequent meals increase satiety, especially if these are high in proteins. This type of meals will help you feel fuller longer. This is especially helpful if you are going on a fast in a few hours after eating.

On a fast, you do not eat anything. That is ideal. For some, 16 hours of 0 calories may be quite a challenge. Intermittent fasting is not that strict. It does not require absolute zero intake during the fasting periods. You may eat during the fast periods, but not as much as in regular eating. Remember, you may eat, but in limited amounts and from within a narrowed list of foods.

Water

This is actually a must when you are in a fast. You absolutely have to drink water. It is critical to drink large amounts of water for many reasons. First, during a fast, you will stimulate several cellular processes that will produce wastes and by-products. It is crucial to eliminate these soon to prevent accumulation within the tissues, which can result to unpleasant symptoms.

Drinking water during a fast helps curb hunger and fight cravings. Most often, when we feel hungry, we are actually thirsty. This is a helpful trick to stave off hunger. When you drink water, your stomach expands - much like when you eat food. The expansion of the stomach muscles will trigger certain stretch receptors that will send a message to the brain. The message will tell the brain to stop feeling or thinking of hunger. Nice trick, huh?

Another good trick is to add certain calorie-free herbs and spices in water with natural appetite-suppressive effects. Add a pinch of cinnamon to your drinking water to combat hunger and cravings. You may also infuse lemon slices to water to suppress hunger and cravings further. Not just that, these add-ons can help in detoxifying your body, taking your fast further.

Tea or Coffee (black)

This is the wildcard for the fast periods. Some IF practitioners take a cup of coffee or tea in the morning to help them extend their fast until their first meal of the day around lunchtime.

A few studies on coffee found that a cup in the morning can increase your body's fat burning potential. Black coffee has been demonstrated to help in curbing hunger in the morning. On the IF, black coffee can boost the fat burning process.

When taking tea or coffee, black is the way to go. You get the full goodness of various active compounds. Adding sugar and/or cream will provide calories in the body that can break your fast.

Green tea is also an acceptable drink in the morning to help you get through. It also has a lot of health benefits, including increased metabolism, better energy and even cancer prevention.

Gum (?)

No. some people on a fast report that chewing sugar-free gum helped them through the 16-hour fast. However, this is not recommended. Some artificial sweeteners in gum can be converted into sugar by the digestive system. These sugars can turn into calories and break your fast. In addition, some gum ingredients may be bad for health and upset the balance of healthy gut bacteria.

Foods to eat in between fasts

This is also known as "what to eat during the window period". This is one of the best points in the 8:16 intermittent fasting diet. You can eat whatever you want. Yes, it does not require complicated food lists or fancy food preparations.

However, if you want get amazing results in the soonest possible time, you have to be smart on food choices in between fasts.

One problem about most of the foods we eat is that they contain too much calories with little nutritional value. Foods made of highly processed ingredients like refined flour, refined sugar and high fructose corn syrup (HCFS) make up most of our diets.

These kinds of foods make it difficult to achieve energy balance in the body. Eat more veggies and meats, instead. These are low in calories but very filling. Vegetables, for instance, are great at making you feel full longer, but they have low calorie content. If you eat 2 cups of vegetables, you will be eating a lot and will feel full for hours. The calories are still low even with the larger servings.

Chapter 12:
Training While on the 8:16 Diet

Aside from the calorie intake, you also need to consider increasing your activity level. What you did in the earlier part of this chapter is to make an honest assessment. Sure, you are now living a sedentary lifestyle. Do you stop there and just eat less? You perform light activity and now you are going on a fast diet. Is that enough to keep you healthy and achieve the weight and body you want?

IF goes beyond merely not eating for the most part of the day. Exercise is also part of the 8:16 intermittent fasting diet. This fasting method takes advantage of the hormonal processes triggered by this state. It also takes advantage of the muscles' increased receptiveness to insulin. This receptiveness means that the muscle cells allow more glucose inside. When more glucose enters the cells, more energy is available. That means the muscles can do more and work harder. This is a vital component if you want to build lean muscles while also maintaining fat loss.

High intensity training is one of the best workouts that will assist in building lean muscles in no time. *Perform this a few times each week during your fasted state.*

On the days that you have scheduled to train, pay more attention to what you eat. This is another component needed to build lean muscles and keep fat loss going hours even after training. Aim to have 2 to 3 meals composed of veggies, proteins (i.e., healthy meats) and carbohydrates on that day. Your largest meal should be right after the training session.

On your non-exercise days, what you eat also matters. Aim to eat 2 to 3 meals composed of veggies, proteins (i.e., meats) and healthy fats.

Foods must be fresh and organic. Limit processed foods to a bare minimum. Supplements are also not advisable. It is still best to allow your body's own hormonal processes and muscle responsiveness to work to create the lean, sculpted look you want.

Chapter 13:
Benefits and Concerns of the 8:16 IF Diet

Your basic goal to get anything good with this diet is to create an energy balance. To get this:

Energy Balance = Calories Out vs Calories In

Your body composition is a result of how you balance energy. That balance will determine weight loss, gain or maintenance.

Most people find it difficult to keep this balance. More calories get in than what the body can use up. The excess is converted into fat then stored. This process gets repeated day after day. This will lead to weight gain and the many problems that come with it - obesity, insulin resistance, diabetes, heart diseases... the list goes on.

With a scheduled eating window (as it is referred to in this diet), you get to be more conscious of when to eat. You can set a limit on how you eat, too.

With the limited eating period, you become more conscious of what you eat. It would be natural to choose foods that will satisfy you and keep you full because you have to be wise if you do not want to be miserable and starve during the entire 16-hour fast. This stricter schedule will make it easier to control calorie intake and attain energy balance.

For beginners, the 16-hour fast may be daunting. It can be a scary thought to go that long without eating, but it does not have to be that way. With proper scheduling, right preparation, smart planning and the determination to keep at it, you will soon see the amazing results of all that hard work.

Main Benefits of the 8:16 IF Diet

The main attractive benefit of this IF diet is getting Wolverine-like pecs. Your massive muscles are not just for show with this diet. The power of the muscles you build in this diet matches the amazing bulk and form.

Aside from that, research on this diet demonstrated a few more benefits. You get great form with better health. The 8:16 IF diet can give you these benefits:

- Lower risk for certain cancers
- Lower risk for having heart diseases
- Promote longer life span
- Better lipid profile
- Lower cholesterol levels
- Improve energy levels
- Promote better organ function
- Reduced cravings for unhealthy foods
- Better cognitive functioning
- Improvement in overall health status
- Better cellular response to insulin
- Increase in fat loss

Concerns about the 8:16 IF diet

There are many ways to make it easier for you to adapt the 8:16 diet, but there are also a few concerns.

One major concern about this is not having the energy to do the things you need to do. For example, if your last meal was last night at 6PM, will you have the energy to do all the things you need to do if you skip breakfast and eat at 12 noon?

Compare how you perform when you eat breakfast, when you take a morning snack and when you skip breakfast. When you eat breakfast, you will feel a slump in your energy level by mid-morning. Your solution is to reach for a quick snack like a sandwich, a cookie or a cup of coffee. By lunchtime, you are hungry again. By mid-afternoon, you will again feel sluggish. You eat snack around dinnertime.

Try skipping breakfast. Sure, the first day may not be fun, but continue doing it for a few days and you will notice a huge difference. On the first day or two, you will feel irritable about not having to eat breakfast. Observe your energy levels. Yes, you are restless and irritable because you will most likely think about food. Consider how your energy level is. The usual mid-morning slump will lessen, if not, totally go away 1-2 days on this diet.

Some people are also concerned about getting ravenous by the time they eat at 11 AM. This is another major concern about the fasting diet. If you do not eat for 16 hours, the question is will you be priming your body to eat a lot once you are in the window period. The idea is that you have been so hungry that once you are allowed to eat, you will be overeating.

No amount of explanation will be enough to convince people that this will not be a huge hurdle on the 8:16 IF diet. We do feel ravenous if we went a few hours without eating. For example, we ate breakfast at 7AM and we are supposed to eat lunch at 12 noon. If we can't eat at that schedule, we feel really hungry. By the time 2PM rolls in and we finally get a chance to eat, of course, we will be eating a lot. This happens a lot of times when we become too busy with stuff and we eat late lunch.

Let us calculate how many hours has lapsed between breakfast at 7AM and late lunch at 2PM. That will be 7 hours. It is really difficult for some people to go more than 3 hours without eating or drinking anything. This is because we have been training our bodies to rely on recently consumed foods for the energy we need for the next few hours.

The hunger you feel is amplified by your psychological state. Yes, you are hungry but not THAT hungry. Your seemingly insatiable appetite often stems from feelings of deprivation - a psychological state or emotional state, which influences your hunger and eating experience.

Try this little experiment. This is not an IF, just a little experiment to see the difference of real and perceived hunger. Eat breakfast at your usual schedule. At any time you feel hungry during the morning, drink a glass of water. Keep doing this until 2PM, when you will eat your late lunch. Observe how you feel a few minutes after drinking water. Chances are, water has reduced your physical hunger pangs but your mind is still preoccupied with food.

Once you are in front of food by 2PM, you do not feel really ravenous but your mind is driving to stuff yourself. You do not really feel hungry but there is that part of your mind, which says finally, you can eat and eat you will.

Who should NOT follow the 8:16 IF Diet?

Intermittent Fasting can work for anyone. It can help anyone get healthy, lose weight and build lean muscles. However, there are a few exceptions. These exceptions are mainly for safety and health reasons. There are certain current health conditions that may worsen when you enter long fasting periods.

Sleep deprived or stressed

People who are experiencing high stress levels for quite a long time are not good candidates for long fasting periods. These also include those who are sleep-deprived. Sleep deprivation and chronic high stress levels take a huge toll on health. Add fasting periods and the body will be subjected to extremely high strain. This can seriously deplete the body's capability to compensate and keep the organs working, further leading to a host of serious, potentially fatal conditions. There can be accelerated cell aging and death, accumulation of toxins, reduced immunity, and slowing of metabolism and organ functioning.

It is advisable to address stress and sleep deprivation first before going in the IF lifestyle.

Sugar or food addict

If you have an addiction to sugar or a certain food, fasting will become especially difficult. You will experience intensified cravings. If you are trying to wean off sugar, then fasting may cause you to relapse. There is a huge possibility that you will gorge on high sugar foods during the eating window. It is better to find other ways to deal with sugar addiction.

Medication

The actions of certain medications are affected by conditions in the body. Adjustments in dosages may be necessary. If you are taking medications for any health condition, inform your doctor about your plan in following the IF diet. Discuss with your doctor first before jumping into the IF life.

Pregnant and breastfeeding women, children

These people have high nutritional requirements for various metabolic and growth needs. Pregnant women need to eat to provide for the nutritional needs of the baby. Prolonged fasting states in pregnant women can lead to weakness and some potential complications like poor fetal growth.

For breastfeeding women, long fasting periods are also not recommended. They need to eat because they have to retain a good supply of nutrients for breast milk production. They also need energy to replenish what they lost during the milk production process and the breastfeeding sessions. This stage can be really taxing on a woman's energy.

Children are at a stage of rapid growth and development. They have high nutritional requirements to fuel growth spurt and the maturation of their various organs. This is not the time to force their bodies into relying on fat stores during fasted states. It is still better for children to eat nutritious foods whenever they are hungry.

Chapter 14:
What is Dry Fasting?

Dry fasting is one of the newest, recently popular health trends these days. An increasing number of people are embracing dry fasting as an effective way to improve health.

Research shows that going on a dry fast helps you to lose excess weight, repair damaged tissue, regenerate old cells, and fight premature aging. It promotes healthy brain functioning by helping the brain produce new neurons.

Aside from generally healing your body and making it stronger and more energy-efficient, dry fasting also has mental and emotional benefits. It clears your mind. It energizes your spirit. It has anti-aging effects that make you look and feel young and age gracefully and beautifully.

What is a Dry Fast?

When you go on a dry fast, you abstain from both food and water for a certain period of time. The body uses stored food and water to keep you going during this time.

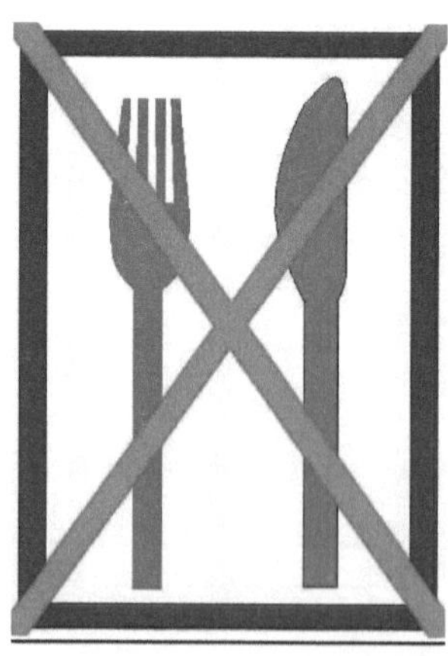

Types of Dry Fasting

<u>There are several ways to go on a dry fast.</u>

•Intermittent dry fasting

This type of dry fasting sets a time window for eating and fasting during the day. Experts in diet and nutrition see this approach as ideal. You get the chance to refuel your body before you start the next day's fast. You get the benefits that result from dry fasting without risking your health.

When you go on an intermittent dry fast, you get to decide when to eat and when to fast.

When you go on a 16/8 intermittent dry fast, you abstain from eating and drinking for 16 hours. You are allowed to eat and drink during the 8-hour window.

When you go on a 20/4 intermittent dry fast, you abstain from food and drink for 20 hours. You are allowed to take food and drink during the 4-hour window.

The RIF or Ramadan Intermittent Fasting that the Muslims practice during Ramadan takes off from this form of fast. Muslims take one meal before sunrise, abstain from food and drink during the hours before sunset (18-20 hours), and take diner before retiring for the night.

•Prolonged dry fasting

Prolonged dry fasting is going without eating and drinking for longer than 24 hours.

People who study diet and nutrition don't recommend this approach.

Fasting for extreme periods of time can result in severe health complications and, in some instances, even death.

The human body is 70% water, suggesting that water is necessary for survival.

You can probably go without taking any food for several weeks. It takes about a month before severe symptoms of starvation set in.

It is different with water. Most people can go without water for 3 days at most. After that, they are likely to be so severely dehydrated that survival is at risk.

There are reports of people meeting accidents in the great outdoors and having to go without water for about 8 days before being rescued. Most of them ate snow and drank their urine in order to survive. Very few barely made it out alive; and among these few, almost everybody went through serious health complications as a result of the experience.

Going on a prolonged dry fast is not advisable. Going without water for a long-drawn-out period can do more harm than good to your health.

Your organs need water to function optimally. Depriving them of water for far longer than necessary can impair them. It is better to keep a dry fast short. Besides, you can enjoy the advantages of dry fasting without taking things to the extreme.

If you want to make dry fasting a part of your lifestyle -- and enjoy the benefits associated with it, you can alternate dry fasts with days where you eat normally. This way, you give your body time to recover from the stress of having to go without food and water.

•Absolute dry fast

When you go on an absolute dry fast, you eliminate any contact with water. You don't brush your teeth, wash, or bathe. You don't touch water at all.

Research shows that the absolute dry fast does not have any additional advantage when compared to the intermittent dry fast. If anything, it may even add to the sense of discomfort or unease that usually comes with fasting.

Chapter 15:
Most Frequently Asked Questions

What is vinegar?

The dictionary defines vinegar as "sour wine" or "a sour liquid obtained by acetic fermentation of dilute alcoholic liquids and used as a condiment or preservative."

How is vinegar made?

Vinegar is made by two distinct biological processes, both the result of the action of harmless microorganisms (yeast and "Acetobacter") that turn sugars (carbohydrates) into acetic acid. Many of our favorite foods involve some type of bacteria in their production – from cheese and yogurt to wine, pickles and chocolate. The first process is called alcoholic fermentation and occurs when yeasts change natural sugars to alcohol under controlled conditions. In the second process, a group of bacteria (called "Acetobacter") converts the alcohol portion to acid. This is the acetic, or acid fermentation, that forms vinegar. Proper bacteria cultures are important; timing is important; and fermentation should be carefully controlled.

What is vinegar made from?

Although acetic acid is the primary constituent of vinegar aside from water, acetic acid is not vinegar. Vinegar contains many vitamins and other compounds not found in acetic acid such as riboflavin, vitamin B-1 and mineral salts from the starting material that impart vinegar with its distinct flavor.

Are there formal standards for vinegar?

Vinegar can be made from any fruit, or from any material containing sugar.

Since vinegar can be made from anything with sugar, there are probably too many different types to count made in countries throughout the world. Each country may use starting materials native to their area and tailored to the specific tastes of the region.

Typical retail varieties of vinegar include white distilled, cider, wine (white and red), rice, balsamic, malt and sugar cane. Other, more specialized types include banana, pineapple, raspberry, flavored and seasoned (e.g., garlic, tarragon).

The following varieties of vinegar are classified by a United States Food and Drug Administration (FDA) Compliance Policy Guide for labeling purposes according to their starting material and method of manufacturing:

Cider vinegar or apple vinegar is made from the two-fold fermentation of the juices of apples. Vinegar can be made from other fruits such as peaches and berries with the labels describing starting materials.

Wine vinegar or grape vinegar is made from the two-fold fermentation of the juice of grapes.

Malt vinegar, made by the two-fold fermentation of barley malt or other cereals where starch has been converted to maltose.

Sugar vinegar, made by the two-fold fermentation of solutions of sugar syrup or molasses.

Spirit or distilled vinegar, made by the acetic fermentation of dilute distilled alcohol.

Blended vinegar made from a mixture of spirit vinegar and cider vinegar is considered a combination of the products that should be labeled with the product names in the order of predominance. It is also the product made by the two-fold fermentation of a mixture of alcohol and cider stock.

Rice or rice wine vinegar (although not part of FDA's Compliance Policy Guide) has increased in popularity over the past several years and is made by the two-fold fermentation of sugars from rice or a concentrate of rice without distillation. Seasoned rice or rice wine vinegars are made from rice with the "seasoning" ingredients noted on the label.

Balsamic vinegar (also not a part of FDA's Compliance Policy Guide) continues to grow in market share and "traditional" and "commercial" forms are available. The products are made from the juice of grapes, and some juice is subjected to an alcoholic and subsequent acetic fermentation and some to concentration or heating. See the "Today's Vinegar" section of the website for more information regarding Traditional and Commercial Balsamic Vinegar.

If you attempt to make vinegar at home, we are sure you'll develop an appreciation for the difficulty of this ancient art and science. Be careful. While homemade vinegar can be good for dressing salads and general purpose usage, its acidity may not be adequate for safe use in pickling and canning. Unless you are certain the acidity is at least four percent, don't pickle or can with it.

What is "Mother"?

"Mother" of vinegar will naturally occur in vinegar products as the result of the vinegar bacteria itself. Mother is actually cellulose (a natural carbohydrate which is the fiber in foods like celery and lettuce) produced by the harmless vinegar bacteria. Today, most manufacturers pasteurize their product before bottling to prevent these bacteria from forming "mother" while sitting on the retail shelf.

After opening, you may notice "mother" beginning to form. Vinegar containing "mother" is not harmful or spoiled. Just remove the substance by filtering and continue to enjoy the product.

How long does vinegar last?

The Vinegar Institute conducted studies to find out and confirmed that vinegar's shelf life is almost indefinite. Because of its acid nature, vinegar is self-preserving and does not need refrigeration. White distilled vinegar will remain virtually unchanged over an extended period of time. And, while some changes can be observed in other types of vinegars, such as color changes or the development of a haze or sediment, this is only an aesthetic change. The product can still be used and enjoyed with confidence.

Is Acetic Acid the same thing as vinegar?

A. No. The United States Food & Drug Administration (FDA) recognizes that diluted acetic acid is not vinegar, indicating that it is:

"misleading if the labeling of a food in which acetic acid is used implies or suggests that the food contains or was not prepared with vinegar. Acetic acid should not be substituted for vinegar in pickled foods, which consumers customarily expect to be prepared with vinegar."

Vinegar has been around for more than 10,000 years, and is one of the few products around today that has been in "Grandma's Kitchen" for centuries. The fermentation of natural sugars to alcohol and then secondary fermentation of alcohol to vinegar is the simple process by which vinegar is made. On the other hand, acetic acid is generally obtained by chemical synthesis of fossil fuel hydrocarbons.

Does vinegar have calories or fat?

Most vinegars contain insignificant amounts of some or all of the mandatory nutrients required in nutrition labeling.

Nutrition labeling is not required if the product contains insignificant amounts of all of the following components (calories, total fat, saturated fat, trans fats, cholesterol, sodium, total carbohydrate, dietary fiber, sugars, protein, vitamin A, vitamin C, calcium and iron) as outlined in the Chapter 21, Section 101.9(j)(4) of the United States Food & Drug Administration's (FDA) Code of Federal Regulations. Most vinegars have less than 3 calories per tablespoon and no fat. Seasoned vinegars may contain more calories due to the added ingredients. Check the label of your favorite vinegar product to determine the nutrition information for that product.

How strong is the vinegar you can buy at retail?

The strength of vinegar is measured by the percent of acetic acid present in the product. All vinegar sold in the United States at the retail level should be at least 4% acidity as mandated by the United States Food & Drug Administration (FDA). Typical white distilled vinegar is at least 4% acidity and not more than 7%. Cider and wine vinegars are typically slightly more acidic with approximately 5-6% acidity.

How can vinegar clean my counters and flavor my pickles?

The acid in vinegar cuts through the grease and germs on your counter tops and is also the ingredient that makes your favorite pickles so tart and safe to eat by inhibiting bacteria and mold. See the "Uses and Tips" section of the website for other ideas for using this versatile product.

What is cleaning vinegar?

A. It is the position of The Vinegar Institute that products labeled as "cleaning vinegar" must contain vinegar.

Products marketed and labeled as "cleaning vinegar" should have vinegar listed in the ingredient statement rather than acetic acid to be assured that the contents are in fact vinegar. Cleaning vinegars should be at a higher strength than table vinegar (i.e., greater than 5% acidity).

Acetic acid is not vinegar.

Vinegar has been around for more than 10,000 years, and is one of the few products around today that has been in "Grandma's Kitchen" for centuries. The fermentation of natural sugars to alcohol and then secondary fermentation of alcohol to vinegar is the simple process by which vinegar is made. On the other hand, acetic acid is generally obtained by chemical synthesis of fossil fuel hydrocarbons

Consumers associate vinegar with natural and environmentally-friendly. Vinegar is well-recognized as a natural ingredient used in cleaning products and for use in lawn/garden applications, which is evidenced by the plethora of "green" tips using vinegar that are available.

Summary Conclusion

Apple cider vinegar is a wonderful elixir. Including it in your daily diet can be very easy. So welcome health, elegance, and strength with as little as a teaspoon of this incredible fluid a day into your life. There's no part of your body excluded from experiencing the amazing effects of apple cider vinegar, practically from the top to toe, inside and outside; if you use it daily, your body will enjoy something tasty.

The ACV is a product readily available that can be easily incorporated into meals. Large-scale work has shown its beneficial properties as a whole material, as well as the strengths of acetic acid and chlorogenic acid in the individual components. ACV can help control blood glucose and lipids, weight loss, and obesity, and can, therefore, be useful for treating type 2 diabetes. Although there is no work directly comparing acetic acid and ACV, ACV as a whole may be more active than acetic acid alone. Consumption of the' vinegar mom' can also improve beneficial effects relative to the lack of this element of ACV. It has been shown that the ACV production method alters the ACV components, which can, in turn, affect the beneficial qualities. To determine the extent of the influence of the production method, further research may be useful here. Yes, ACV use may help control type 2 diabetes.

There are NUMEROUS published studies done on ACV and it's weight loss effects, cleansing action and overall health benefits for people all over the world for a long time.

Try reading some of these published articles on any of the major medical search engines displaying most of the published research articles on ACV and it's health effects. ACV is one of the most overlooked, under-rated health supplements available at such a low cost and almost every main grocer or health supplement store sells it.

The End..or Is It a New Beginning?

www.ingramcontent.com/pod-product-compliance
Lightning Source LLC
Chambersburg PA
CBHW051222250726
48655CB00006B/2550